AZTHETIKS INNOVATION X-TREME

A BODYBUILDER'S GUIDE FOR MUSCLE BUILDING TRANSFORMATION

I0101760

ROB NITER

WWW.AZTHETIKS-INNOVATION.COM

Azthetiks Innovation X-Treme

(A Bodybuilder's Guide for Muscle Building Transformation)

by

Rob Niter

Disclaimer

Copyright © 2015

US Copyright Office: Registration# TXu001990876

All Rights Reserved.

No part of this eBook can be transmitted or reproduced in any form including print, electronic, photocopying, scanning, mechanical or recording without prior written permission from the author.

While the author has taken utmost efforts to ensure the accuracy of the written content, all readers are advised to follow information mentioned herein at their own risk. The author cannot be held responsible for any personal or commercial damage caused by misinterpretation of information. All readers are encouraged to seek professional advice when needed.

About Azthetiks Innovation X-Treme

This book is specially written for bodybuilders, fitness fanatics or someone who seeks a healthy lifestyle change. If you are unsure of your training technique or workout routine, this book can help you maximize your inner potential and aid you in excelling in the art of body transformation. If you have a thousand questions in the back of your mind about mass development and muscle building, read ahead. This book was specially written to help clear your doubts and provide you with comprehensive and accurate knowledge about bodybuilding. If you think your workout routine or training program is ineffective and nothing works for you, this book can help you get a good start. I have discussed several topics in this book that I think will be most beneficial. They are:

- The basics of mass development in body building
- Workout routines and programs
- Nutrition
- Supplements
- Motivation

In this book, I have also discussed some common variables and problems that a bodybuilder faces frequently. I hope this will help you solve your challenges and answer those questions which you are too afraid to or shy to ask anyone else.

Table of Contents

Table of Contents

Chapter#1: Introduction to Bodybuilding

I have been in the fitness industry for a very long time. I often meet people who are looking for a secret formula or a magic supplement to gain muscle mass rapidly. I always tell them what I am going to tell you. Bodybuilding is an art. Treat your body with respect and you will most definitely see results. Using natural and healthy techniques is the first step to gaining a healthy mass volume.

You cannot rush the process of building muscles. It's not magic. I have strived for countless years to gain extensive knowledge and experience in the field of health and fitness. I am proud that after so many years of research and practice, I am able to impart my knowledge so that others can benefit from my hard work and avoid the mistakes a beginner makes. It is extremely rewarding and important for me to see people who have transformed their lives from my workout routines, motivation and inspiration.

I have read the conventional articles in the magazine, telling people how and what they should eat, train and even feel; which is often incorrect and gives off a negative vibe. The media has plunged our generation into a self defeating agenda of eating less and training more. I encourage my trainees to ignore the so called "secrets of a healthy life" and focus on setting an achievable goal.

Don't fall prey to the concepts of quick weight loss, cleanses, crash diets and quick fixes. They all sound so delectable, don't they? But all of these fitness advices defeat the purpose of a healthy life. The only thing you can achieve by these solutions is a miserable and exhaustive life. There is no point in trying to eat fewer calories to lose those extra pounds. It will only make you frustrated. Try and focus on what you want to achieve. Set a goal. Train for the body you want. This is where everything will change for you.

Changing your routine is not the only precedent of a healthy lifestyle. Being physically, mentally and psychologically prepared is also very important. I have seen people who start with a bang and stay on the right path of muscle building, but eventually, they fall victim to the burn-out syndrome. If you want to start on the path of building your body mass, make sure that you are in a motivated state of mind. Follow discussion boards, relate to the people who are on the same path as you. In short, do anything to keep your motivation and inspiration level at the top.

What Is Bodybuilding?

Bodybuilding is the art of developing the muscles in your body by weight training, exercising and strength training. As a fitness trainer and pro bodybuilder, I am often asked this question. In light of my experience and expertise, I define bodybuilding as the balance of a good training program, rest and proper nutrition. It is an amazing physical activity which is beneficial, not just for your body but also for your mind. I have seen numerous people fight depression, anxiety and even insomnia by completely giving their lifestyle a healthier makeover.

The word bodybuilding basically tells you everything you need to know. It implies the basic meaning of this sport. Don't confuse bodybuilding with other fitness fads. It's not like a crash exercise regime that will help you lose weight before the bikini season. Bodybuilding is a lifestyle. In order to be successful at it, you will need to incorporate it completely into your life and make subsequent changes and sacrifices that it demands. Hence, bodybuilding is a way of living that can provide a routine and structure to your life.

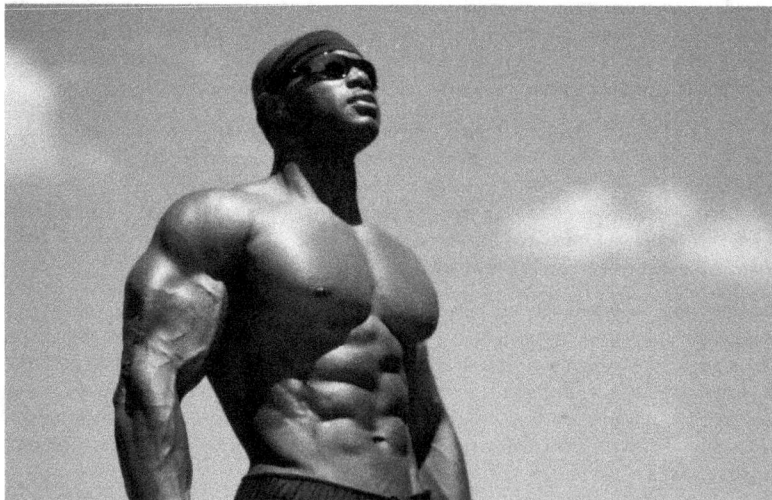

It Is a Lifestyle

There are many people who are intimidated with the concept of building muscles. They see the world of bodybuilding as a fear of having to dedicate a significant amount of time and energy to obtain their bodybuilding goals; which will take them away from their social and family life. Let me ease your mind. Bodybuilding is all about integrating a healthy outlook into your lifestyle.

Moderation and a well-rounded approach works best when you are working towards your goal of a better physique. However, bodybuilding is not an overnight transformation, but rather a process. Keeping that in mind, it's important to understand that it's not about being the biggest and strongest individual around. It is a learning and growth process during which a bodybuilder improves self.

What Is A Bodybuilder?

Discipline and dedication are important tools that can help you become a hardcore competitive bodybuilder. People often want to put a label on body types and fitness achievements. They often ask me what a bodybuilder is. Is it the amount of weight they can lift? Or is it just dependent on how buff and sculpted they physically look? They often associate the well-oiled heavily muscled bodies of bodybuilders with mass. They are not the only types of bodybuilders there are.

Athletes and individuals that change their lifestyles and fitness and nutrition details to improve their body and mass definition are all bodybuilders in my eyes. There are no specific exercises or the number of gym hours that will include you in the bodybuilder category. Every individual has a different body type which we will discuss in this chapter. This prevents the possibility of a ready-made program or formula that would work for everyone. With the right customized fitness program designed by me, you can achieve your dream body.

Natural bodybuilding

I always tell people to stop trying to find a short cut in mass development, because there is no magic formula. Many synthetic and chemical supplements manufacturers have blurred the distinction between the legal supplements and harmful steroids. This is where natural bodybuilding comes in. Contrary to popular belief, natural bodybuilding does exist. I am a living example that you don't need steroids and illegal supplements to maximize your muscle definition to accelerate your body transformation.

A natural bodybuilder understands and respects the limits of their body. It is important to adhere to the genetic limitations of your body and not push it towards goals that are impossible and unattainable. It is sad to see when people who are new to mass development freely ask the question of "how many drugs I have to take?" You cannot ignore the underlying and long-term effects of these chemicals on your health. This book will help you get acquainted with the fact that you can muscle-up without relying on the harmful chemicals and steroids.

Important Facts about Mass Building

Gaining mass is more difficult for people who are initially skinny or have less meat on their bones. I see people who eat all the time and have nothing to show for it. Fast metabolism can be a curse when it comes to mass development. However, I have compiled a list of some facts that can help you to gain mass weight if nothing seems to work for you.

1) Training Duration

It doesn't matter which training program or fitness regime you follow, keep the duration under 1 to 1.5 hours. Rather than increasing the time of your workout, gradually increase your intensity. I have often emphasized on the importance of high intensity. Working for more than one hour will not help you to reap any benefits; rather it will cause all kinds of hormonal damages. Therefore, work harder, not longer.

2) Consistent Eating Habits

People who cannot seem to gain any muscle mass no matter how efficiently they train should look into their eating timetable. Inconsistencies and irregularities in eating can hinder your chances of gaining any weight. People with low body mass are often pre-programmed with a fast metabolism which quickly burns the consumed calories. My suggestion is to break down your meal pattern into groups of 5-7 and space them apart every 2-3 hours. In this way, your body will have a constant supply of calories and nutrients to metabolize, which will increase your prospect of mass gain.

3) Caloric Surplus

I have seen countless cases where people eat a lot and don't seem to gain any muscle mass. The problem is that they are unaware of the concept of calorie surplus. It doesn't matter how much you eat, but rather, what you eat. If you are unable to gorge on large amounts of food, focus on eating high caloric food. The high content in calories will help you with your gains. If you are still unsure about what to eat, read ahead. The proper nutrient intake has been discussed in detail in the last chapter of this book.

Identifying Your Body Type

The first step to program a specialized workout for you is to know your body type. Each body is created differently. Before starting a workout regime and nutrition program, it is inherent that you find out your body type and train according to that. There are basically three types of bodies. Find out which one you possess and determine your diet and workout routine based on that.

- Ectomorph

This body type is characterized by the prevalence of body fat. An ectomorph will seem to be much thinner than they really are. They have narrow hips and clavicles, long limbs, small wrist/ankle bones and stringy muscle bellies.

- Mesomorph

Mesomorphs have well defined and developed muscle structure. They are intrinsically characterized by their wide clavicles, narrow waist, long well defined bellies and small, thin joints. This is the ideal body type that can withstand the added amount of weight without looking heavy or bulky. Their bodies look well-proportioned even when they put on a little extra weight.

- Endomorph

Endomorphs are naturally bulky with a thick rib cage, wide hips and clavicles, thick joints and short limbs. Their bodies look heavy even when they are ripped.

Can Bodybuilding Help You?

Exercise is good for you. In fact, it is the miracle cure that we have used for centuries to fight against diseases like heart attacks, strokes, diabetes, arthritis and even an early death. People, who are physically active, reap the benefits of a longer life than those who are not. It has been recommended by doctors for decades as an ingredient to sustaining a healthier life.

1) It Can Help You Combat Diseases

We all know is the importance of exercise. It doesn't matter what type you indulge in. Cardio exercises increase your heart rate and help burn fat by melting the unwanted calories in our body. But that's only a small part of the equation. If you really want to get into the whole fitness spirit, strength training and mass development is inherent. It can prevent the slow deterioration of muscles that comes naturally with old age. The solution is this! Increase your muscle mass and develop stronger and lithe muscles to combat the problems associated with muscle and bone loss.

People who don't train and live a sedentary life often find themselves on the cusp of old age when their bones are riddled with arthritis and their connective tissues loose definition. Muscle building helps prevent that. It can help you to increase your bone density, ease arthritis pain and cut your risk of further injuries. I have seen old people make excuses that they cannot build their muscle mass because they are too old. It's a misconception that is hindering them from achieving a better life.

2) It Can Help You Lose Weight

We must not forget the advantages of muscle building in weight loss. It can assist you to achieve your dream body which is lithe, shapelier and trim. I've come across several females who have been misguided in the past on the subject of muscle building. I hear things like, "if I lift weights, I will look manly" or "the squats will make my butt look too big". Males are not too far behind. They say stuff like "I want definition and don't want a bulky body, so I can just use light weights and high reps to get cuts, right?"

These are the kind of mythical and incorrect beliefs that I educate my clients about. I repeatedly tell them why muscle building is good. These fitness and training myths have their basis in a lot of fitness books and training customs. What's really important is to understand that they are just myths. Muscle building will prevent excess weight gain. When you engage in an intense training routine, it can boost your energy levels and endurance. It helps to deliver oxygen and nutrients to your tissues and aid in the better distribution of blood to the cardiovascular system.

3) It Can Ameliorate the Skeletal Muscles

It is an inherent part of the muscle building phenomena. Mass development helps to preserve and increase the existing levels of skeletal muscles in your body. People are often confused about what a skeletal muscle is. They are basically the muscles surrounding the skeleton and attached by bundles of collagen fibers known as tendons. They are active metabolically and the more calories you burn with strength training, the more emphasis on the recovery process you will require.

It's not rocket science that building skeletal muscles give your body a toned look and restore and fortifies the bone and tendon ligaments. Having stronger skeleton muscles means that you will live longer and persevere better in the face of any injury. They enhance the quantity of insulin receptors which naturally reduce body fat and assist in fat loss.

4) Help Improve Your Sports Performance

Have you ever witnessed an athlete that doesn't have a toned body with an excellent muscle definition? And I am not just talking about athletes into weight training and muscle building sports. They are all familiar with the importance of a good muscle definition and its impact on their performance. If you want to fire up your sports activities, building muscle mass is the best solution. If you want to jump higher, run longer or hit harder, developing a strong muscle definition can maximize your sport's performance. There is no need to blame genetics or your gender, if you have a positive mindset and aspire to be better, success will follow.

Muscle mass building can aid you to focus on the key areas of your sports training. It improves speed, strength and agility and will have a huge impact on the overall performance to make your responsive nerves quick, powerful and continuous. You must keep in mind, that developing muscle mass is not skills training; it is a secondary non-sport training to enhance your sport dynamics and variables.

Can You Build Muscles Without Gaining Fat?

Have you ever faced the situation when your muscle build-up dwindles away when you lower your diet standards? Are you worried that reducing calories will help you to lose muscle definition? Many people face this conundrum. Building muscles while burning fat is not an easy feat, especially when you have a hard task of developing a ripped body and hard sculpted abs. Often, experts confuse the two facts. Most of them will tell you that in order to reach optimum success, you will have to choose between gaining muscles and gaining fat.

However, it is possible to gain muscle without gaining fat. You will need to follow a concise path of dedication and discipline and acute planning. There are several things that aid in burning fat while keeping the muscles in place.

The Right Food

This is a no-brainer. You cannot underestimate the power of a planned nutritional time table. It will make meal planning a little difficult initially, but you can manipulate proteins, carbs and fat while planning your meals and remain strict with the eating guidelines. Without adhering to a strict diet regime, it will be impossible for you to realize your fitness objective of building mass.

Muscles are generally made from protein, constituting amino acids as the building blocks. During or after physical training, your body craves amino acids for restoration and recovery. The human body breaks down the protein into amino acids and uses them for various bodily functions, while the remaining amino acids get converted into other useable molecules by the liver. In order to balance out the protein loss, it is ideal to consume at least 1.5 grams of protein per pound of your bodyweight divided by the total number of meals you are going to have in a single day. Protein should be distributed evenly throughout the day to help better integration. This can ensure optimal muscle mass formation without any increase in fat. If you don't have a steady stream of amino acids in your diet, you may experience tissue loss over time, which is counter-effective for building muscle mass.

Know These Rules for a High Impact Muscle Training

Like every field, body building is a discipline which is surrounded by the speculation of which method works best. These speculations often lead to confusion and frustration which can de-motivate an aspiring bodybuilder. For example, in terms of nutrition, there is a common myth surrounding fats that their omission from the diet can help with a better muscle definition and fat loss. However, that is incorrect. A healthy dose of fats not only aids in muscle formation, but in appropriate ratios, it can improve your health and physical development. Before going down the path of muscle building, you should know these basic rules.

1) Progress towards Heavier Weights

A bodybuilder must understand that the key element to increase muscle mass is to increase the amount of weights gradually. This progression can result directly in the subsequent increase in intensity of the overall workout and ensure that the muscles are subject to enough stress in yielding results.

The first aim of a bodybuilder should be to quantify the repetitions with a certain amount of weight (say 10 repetitions with 25 kilograms weight). Over the next few weeks, that weight should be increased to 27.5 and so on. The goal is to expose the muscles with progressive stress continuously without prolonged breaks or delays. If this process is ruled out, then the workout intensity hits a plateau which will eliminate the body to gain any muscle mass whatsoever.

2) Bulk Up On Protein

It is inherent that you consume at least 1 gram of protein per pound of your bodyweight to ensure that you don't lose muscle mass. If you are subjecting your muscles to great amounts of stress, it is only fair that you treat your body well by maintaining a steady stream of protein in your diet. A high percentage of protein is the second most important thing after training intensity. Timing is also very important in protein consumption. Inconsistency or incorrect meal timings can create imbalance in your metabolism, so stick to a strict schedule and don't miss out on your protein consumption.

3) Get Rest

Giving your body the time to restore and heal is a smart thing to do after a hard and intense workout. Sleep is inherent to protein synthesis and helps the body to mentally and physically recharge for the next training session. If you are not getting enough sleep, you will feel tired and exhausted. Your testosterone and hormonal balances will become disturbed and that will directly affect your next training session.

Respecting your body is very important. At initial stages, lack in sleep can lead your muscles to break down in order to supply glycogen to the brain and other organs. Ideally, I advise you to get at least 7+ hours of sleep per night. Take a warm bath, listen to some music and try to relax and you will have a systemized sleeping pattern in no time.

4) Be Positive

Developing a positive mental attitude will help you to improve your muscle building process. If you approach each workout/training session with a zealous attitude, the quality will certainly improve and you will feel a significant rise in your self-confidence. It is very simple and straightforward. Negative feelings will have a negative impact on your training. It is very important to keep your eye on your goal and try to achieve your expectations by building a relationship between your mind and muscles. When you start visualizing your success and that amazing well-sculpted body, it will bring you to one step closer to your goal.

5) Feel Happy

Stress plays a destructive role. I have seen many people give in to the feeling of anxiety and stress. This usually occurs when people expect to get results magically in a short amount of time and when that doesn't happen, they feel disappointed. Negative stress can produce high amounts of Cortisol in your body. I encourage people to stay away from any stress-inducing variables like smoking, drinking or even lack of sleep. All of these dynamics can cause protein break-down and fat accumulation which is the direct opposite of what a bodybuilder strives for.

6) Consume Fats

Are you aware that fats are actually good for you? Well, not all fats, but some of them. Contrary to the popular belief, fat intake can be productive in muscle building and weight loss. However, it is essential that you consume healthy fats in order to maintain your testosterone levels and energy levels.

7) Avoid Over Exerting Your Body

Many fitness enthusiasts are often plagued with this problem. They push the limits of their bodies, while not understanding that overtraining will destroy any chance of muscle growth (ex. 3+ hours in the gym). It will likely cause muscle regression. A bodybuilder should listen to the warning signs of their body and if presented with pain or discomfort, they should cease or change their current training routine immediately.

8) Educate Yourself

Bodybuilding is not just about joining a gym and lifting weights. There is a whole science behind it. It is highly advisable that you hire a trainer to help you get through the different stages of muscle development. As a bodybuilder, you will have to go through the process of continuous learning and experimentation. Without consulting experienced experts and researching, a bodybuilder will not be able to advance and progress beyond the initial stages of a beginner.

Amateurs spend a lot of time trying to find the "secrets" to improve their mass building aspirations. There is no secret; rather there are tried and tested prerequisites that are fundamentally important to gaining muscle mass. In the next chapter, you will get to know my training routines and exercises which have been evaluated personally by me over the course of many years.

Chapter#2: Workout Routines and Programs

The most important variable in my mass building is the selection of a perfect workout routine and program. Identifying the right plan for working out is crucial for promoting the process of muscle building. A workout routine is basically the exercises that are categorized in a well laid out plan for a person to follow every day. The amount of weight, number of repetitions, order and the type of exercises are all mentioned and explained in an effective workout routine.

However, you should keep in mind that mass building is not an easy task. You need a dedicated workout routine to follow, in order to achieve your goal of consistent muscle building. It will seem complicated and difficult to you at first, but as you get into the habit of muscle training, you will become accustomed to the whole process. At most gyms or training facilities, the available trainers can help you discover the optimum training program based on your body type and goal. I carefully design my workout routines by taking my client's goal, age, fitness level and lifestyle into consideration. As a training expert, I have dedicated my life to finding the perfect combination of cardio and strength training exercises in helping people attain the results they desire.

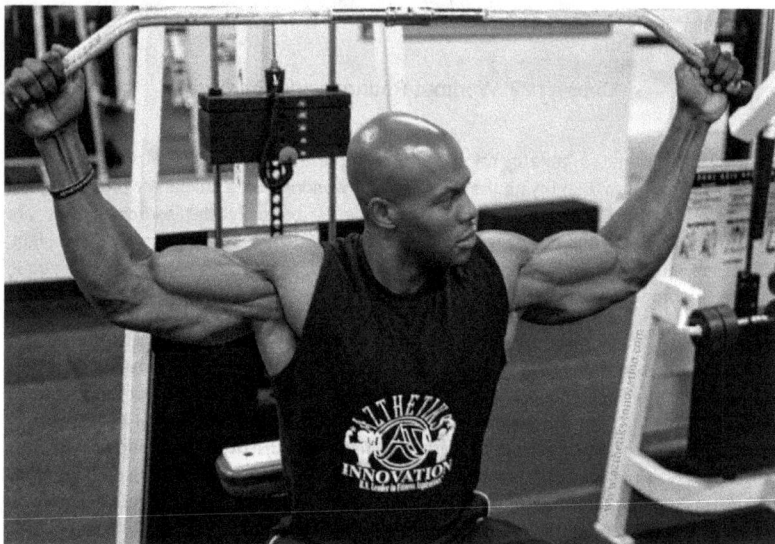

I have seen people without a workout program who complain that they are not seeing any results. A good workout routine that is designed specifically for you will increase your chance of adhering to the routine and achieving success. A balanced workout routine should be carefully followed and monitored to measure the intensity and duration of the workout as well as your adherence to the exercise mode.

When Your Workout Plan Doesn't Work

There are many instances when even a workout plan doesn't yield favorable results. There can be several reasons for that, such as:

1) Ineffective Workout Routine

As I have stated earlier, working out more is not the answer. For bodybuilding, you need to train harder, not longer. And choosing a compatible and right routine is inherent for the realization of your mass building objective. An effective workout routine should be designed to suit your body type, training experience and your desired goal. If you are not seeing results, it means that your workout routine is not designed based on these variables. It will thus, result in a waste of time, energy and motivation without producing results.

2) You Ignore Constructive Feedback

I have seen countless fitness fanatics who lean toward the feedback of inexperienced friends and fellow peers, while ignoring guidance from an experienced trainer or coach. You can learn quite a lot from an experienced individual that has "been there and done that"! Don't discount their feedback. Take their suggestions into consideration. You can learn about resting periods, muscle group arrangement during workout days, isolation and compound exercises and warm up tips. Use their knowledge to maximize the impact of your exercises.

3) Using the Same Workout Routine

The concept of muscle building is based on the body's reaction to stress and intensity. The inability to increase mass ratio can be directly related to the fact that you have not bothered to change the intensity and number of reps for the core exercises in your routine. If the workout routine is not changed periodically, the muscle growth becomes stagnant because the body quickly adapts to the stress amount. If subsequent changes are not made in the workout program, the muscles will not grow in size or strength. It is generally preferable to change your workout routine every 10-12 weeks for maximum results.

4) Bad Exercise Technique

Efficiency is not the only thing that affects your muscle growth and doing the right exercises is not enough. How you do them defines if you will succeed or fail. A bad exercise technique can cause failure or worse, injury. The execution of the exercise in a proper way and with the correct movement will keep the risk of injury at bay. You should keep the reps controlled and perform them with slow and accurate momentum. When you are dealing with weights, don't swing them. Rather, use a full range of motions to control your joint movement.

Is Training Different Than Working Out?

If you are stuck in a time capsule where muscle building is a concern, you need to shake things up to gain maximum results. For some people, nothing seems to work. If the dedication to working out doesn't produce results, the obvious solution is to correct the orientation of goals and training to achieve the desired outcome.

Many people don't understand that there is no difference between training and working out. They are different sides of the same coin and one cannot exist without the other. Working out is not merely showing up at your training facility and going through the prescribed workout routine. In order to realize your goals, you need to train your mind and body. The training part usually takes place outside the gym. Proper nutrition, sleep patterns and your food intake are all part of training your body and changing your lifestyle. Training requires a specific goal and that goal can be achieved by a specific workout program. Result orientation can help you to visualize your objective and establish a performance directed workout for maximum gains.

The next section of this chapter includes several workout routines and programs that can help you increase mass structure and build muscles.

Part 1: Cardio

One of the most challenging parts of designing a workout program is to balance cardio with weight training. A complete workout routine should include a combination of cardiovascular and weight training. The desired goal will determine how the two should be integrated into a program. Taking your objectives into consideration before identifying the perfect balance between cardio and weight training is paramount to overall success.

Identify Your Goals

Finding out your primary goal is pretty straightforward. Ask yourself this question before designing your workout routine. *Are you working out to lose fat, gain muscle or do both?* The cardio training will solely be dependent on the answer to this question.

Your primary goal will provide you with an initial strategy to figure out the correct balance between your weight and cardio training. You will be more successful in achieving your goal when you have a specific objective in mind because there are different processes and techniques for different training processes.

Do You Want To Gain Muscle or Lose Fat?

If you are training to lose body fat, you will need more cardio than a person who is trying to gain muscle mass. To gain optimum fat loss results, do cardio training twice a week, 20 to 30 minutes per session. However, these sessions will yield successful results for muscle gain, only when they are combined with weight training at least 3-6 times a week. Remember, shy away from the scale. If you are gaining muscle and losing fat, you won't see much of a difference in numbers!

Types of Cardio

There are three basic types of cardio training that can have a maximized effect on muscle building if they are done frequently.

1) Low-Intensity Cardio

This includes walking and slow cycling. This type of cardio training can be done almost every day without any extended rest periods. Your body will easily recover from this type of training and will help you to lose fat without any subsequent loss in muscle mass.

2) Moderate-Intensity Cardio

Moderate-intensity cardio include exercises such as jogging and swimming which should be done less frequently as more energy is required for performance and recovery process. If you are trying to lose fat, you can generally partake in moderate-intensity workouts, 6 sessions per week. However, -this amount should be reduced to just 2-3 sessions and no more than 20 to 30 minutes if you are trying to gain muscles.

3) High-Intensity Cardio

If you are looking for fast and great results, high-intensity cardio can help you achieve that. High-intensity cardio exercises such as sprinting and interval training can be done for short periods of time with short rest periods. This type of training is extremely effective for fat loss as it burns a lot of calories within a short time. It also increases your metabolism to a great degree after the workout is finished.

Cardiovascular Workouts

Cardio has been a controversial topic in the bodybuilding community for years. Many people believe that cardio has the ability to sap strength, shrivel up muscles and hinder gains. The most important issue that muscle builders have to deal with everyday is the effect cardio has on muscle growth. Cardio can help with the muscle growth and overall appearance in several ways. So don't discount it!

Cardio and Muscle Recovery

Intensive workout sessions can cause muscle damage which is most commonly known as Delayed Onset Muscle Soreness or DOMS. But feeling sore for a day or two is normal after an intense workout session. Muscle recovery can be a complex process which can be quickened by cardio because it increases the blood flow and helps the body and remove waste.

Cardio and Metabolism

In a perfect scenario, all the nutrients from the food intake should be absorbed into the muscles and none should result in fat accumulation. But each body is different and performs in varying degrees where nutrient absorption is a concern. Some bodies store less fat than others when they overeat, while others store excess amount of calories or lose muscle when they restrict their calorie intake. Knowing your body and how it functions will help you in reaching your max potential.

Hormones like Cortisol and testosterone also affect the metabolism and food absorption in our body. Insulin is another genetic variable that affects the process of food absorption. When you are eating surplus calories to gain muscles, insulin sensitivity can be a beneficial asset because insulin resistance can hinder muscle growth and promote fat storage in your body. Cardio is one of the ways through which you can manipulate the metabolism because it increases insulin sensitivity in a dose dependent manner. This means the more cardio you do, the more improvement you will see.

The Best Time to Do Cardio

There is no cookie cutter formula for specifying the best time to do cardio and it differs from person to person depending upon their body type. But there are a few guidelines that will help you to understand the best time to perform cardio which will produce better results.

1) Cardio in the morning

Doing cardio first thing in the morning, on an empty stomach is a big NO. It's not good for your body and should be avoided at all costs. It can result in muscle loss and loss in energy, which is a body builder's worst nightmare. Most of the trainers emphasize the importance of pre-workout nutrition for this very purpose, because doing cardio on an empty stomach will decrease your performance significantly as you won't have the energy reserves to compliment your workout.

2) Cardio before weight training

This is another thing that should be avoided if you want to gain maximum results from weight training. Cardio before an intense weightlifting can deplete your body's glycogen reserves which are needed to give the muscles an extra push during the last few minutes of your weight session. If you do cardio before the session, the protein synthesis drops to a low level and causes the protein to break up. This drop in protein synthesis negatively affects the body's ability to build muscles.

3) Cardio after weight training

It is preferable to do cardio *after* weight training than before it. The main reason is that weight lifting doesn't diminish your glycogen stores which can be used during the cardio, depending on the intensity and duration of the session. But for a more effective performance and great results, wait for a couple hours after lifting weights to start on your cardio.

Cardiovascular Workouts and Muscle Growth

Nobody is going to argue with the fact that cardio doesn't make you a better lifter. If cardio is used alone, it can help you achieve a lean, muscular and athletic looking body. But when it is combined with weight lifting in the right frequency, it can help you achieve all your muscle building objectives. There are several reasons for that.

First off, having a strong heart is efficient for obvious health reasons. Frequent cardio exercises can have a great impact on your heart's stroke volume, which is basically the heart's ability to pump out blood from the left ventricle. If the heart can pump more blood with less work, it can directly affect the intensity and duration of your cardio sessions and can be advantageous for gaining muscular strength over time.

Second, cardiovascular exercises have a positive effect on your blood vessels. A highly effective heart needs a healthy network of capillaries to perform steady weightlifting and other workout routines. Cardio helps increase the blood flow and volume to the muscles, which is impossible to achieve by weightlifting alone. Cardio also increases the tissue capacity to perform at a higher level and helps it to absorb oxygen and nutrients quickly. As stated previously, it facilitates muscle recovery and clears away metabolites and other waste products from the body.

Energy Enhancement

Bodybuilding or developing muscle mass is the stimulation of mind to produce energy by muscle movement. To move muscles, you need to produce energy which increases the overall energy expenditure. The more energy that you utilize during a workout, the more energy you will have during the rest periods. The key to building muscle mass is to lose fat and build muscles at the same time while increasing energy.

The bottom line is that increased muscle stimulation results in a direct gain in energy expenditure which increases the production of energy in our body. When we move the muscles in the body, we are in effect calling upon our minds to use the latent energy reserves. When our latent energy is ignited, we fire up our bodies to burn more energy for longer periods of times. Cardiovascular exercises are a great example of energy enhancement workouts.

How to Decrease Fatigue?

There are a number of variables in the energy equation. The energy production is partly dependent upon the pre-training activity which should include factors to facilitate your training in an effective way. First, the pre-training activity should provide a physical and mental motivation for you to attack the workout with all your might. This motivation will help you to endure the hard part of the training. Even if you are exerting maximum pressure on yourself during the workout, the endurance from the pre-training motivation will help you complete the workout.

Second, it should provide you with an increased aerobic and anaerobic energy for training by decreasing the central and peripheral fatigue. Third, it should help facilitate a quick and better recovery post-workout.

In addition to proper motivation before the workout, a bodybuilder must keep in mind the importance of decreasing the mental fatigue and stress during the workout. This type of fatigue is called central fatigue and results from the impaired functions of the central nervous system. It has little effect on the muscles, but indirectly, it can lower your ability to perform better. A bodybuilder must take proper steps to increase their neurotransmitter levels to decrease perceived exertion and become more focused and productive during a workout.

Biotin Provides an Energy Boost

Proper motivation is not the only key element in energy enhancement. A little energy boost from biotin will help you to increase efficiency during the training sessions. You must have heard about biotin, as it's a major hair and nail supplement. What you don't know is that biotin plays a huge role in the development of muscles in your body. It has the ability to bind proteins in your body by breaking down the fats, carbohydrates and protein into energy for use. If you are not consuming enough biotin, most of the protein and other nutrients are not being properly utilized. Biotin can help your body to produce energy on the cellular level and its deficiency can cause fatigue and lethargy.

How to Increase and Maintain Energy

There are several ways to increase and maintain your body's energy reserves throughout the day and not just during the training sessions. Some of them are listed below.

1) Recharge your body by getting a good amount of sleep every night.
2) Get out in the sun and get vitamin D from the natural source. The light and the warm rays from the sun produce vitamin D in our body and maintain a consistence cardiac rhythm which plays an important role in energy reservation.

3) Eat consistently throughout the day and don't skip meals. Regular nutrient intake will help you to perform all mental and physical activities with ease. Eat food rich in fiber and natural sugars to provide the energy you need.
4) Keep yourself hydrated at all times. As we know, life cannot exist without water. During a workout, a person loses about 4-8 cups of water through sweating. If you don't consume enough water, the lack of water can cause you to feel dizzy, nauseous and light headed. So drink up as this vital nutrient makes up roughly 80% of our body!
5) Consume caffeine rich foods. Caffeine is the most reliable source of energy and is easily available. It is a fast acting substance which can increase your energy and create mental alertness. However, it should only be used as a temporary boost of energy.

The Best Workout to Increase Energy

If you are feeling tired and lethargic, it means that you are suffering from low levels of energy. The good news is that you can increase your energy reserves by incorporating an appropriate training and workout session into your routine. Although it may seem that training more would be a drain on your existing energy reserves, but trust me, these exercises will actually help you to increase your energy levels.

Resistance Training

Resistance training includes different types of training exercises ranging from stretch band workouts to intense weight lifting. You can choose a resistance training exercise based upon your objective. Your goal will also help you determine the intensity of your resistance training. Another great fact about this workout is that it has a direct relationship with metabolism. And as resistance training increases lean muscle mass in your body, the body burns more calories per day which allows you to eat more and develop muscle mass and lose fat at the same time.

Cardiovascular Exercises

Cardio is another type of energy enhancing exercise that increases you heart rate to a significant level in a moderate amount of time which facilitates the body to burn more calories. The immense amount of calorie loss can have a direct impact on fat loss and weight loss. As the body goes through the process of losing fat, it will take less energy to move around and you will feel more energetic.

Heart Rate Training

Heart rate training is basically customizing your workout and training routines based upon the performance of your heart. Heart monitors are an optimum way to achieve this objective. They can help you to lose weight, enhance workout optimization, and increase muscular mass and improve the agility and conditioning of the overall exercise routine.

How Can You Monitor You Heart?

Technology has advanced to an extent where the heart monitor doesn't just measure the heart rate but also perform other activities such as beep at you when you exceed your target exercise range. It can alert you to move faster if you are slowing down unconsciously. Most of the heart rate monitors have a built in function to measure the amount of calories burned and analyze your training sessions. The GPS function can aid you in determining the distance than you ran or traveled.

When you are wearing a heart rate monitor, it will constantly record your vitals like blood pressure, heart beats per minute and calories burned. Even if you don't own a heart rate monitor, you are already sort of heart rate training. The only difference is people with a heart rate monitor can do it in a more definite and precise fashion.

In a nutshell, monitoring your heart rate gives you an advantage of precision and to eliminate subjective and perceived variables. Monitoring your heart rate for different outcomes during HRT is known as training zones which will be discussed later. First, you must know the 2 variables that are used to calculate the training zones. These variables are explained below.

1) Maximum Heart Rate

Most people with a beginner's knowledge about heart rate calculation know that in order to find your maximum heart rate you have to subtract your age from 220. This equation was first introduced in the 1930's and it has no authenticity when it comes to individuals. Every human body is different. You cannot calculate the maximum heart rate of a person without taking into account their health attributes and general lifestyle. The most reliable way to find your maximum heart rate without a monitor is to use the accurate method of lactate threshold (LT).

2) Lactate Threshold

Many of you must be unfamiliar with the term lactate threshold. It is directly related to the lactic acid as the name suggests. When your body is performing at low intensity, the muscles produce lactates which are absorbed by the body. This overall process keeps the lactic acid concentration in the blood low.

However, when you increase the intensity at which your body performs, the body starts producing more lactic acid than it can absorb and its concentration in the blood goes up.

This is the point when the body cannot keep up with the lactate production. This is called the lactate threshold, the highest intensity which can be maintained in a human body for a period of 30 minutes. You will have a different LT for each sport and activity based on the amount of intensity involved in the sport.

How to Find Your Lactic Threshold?

The lactic threshold can be determined by choosing an intensive sport or workout routine that you can perform consistently for at least 30 minutes. Cycling and running are excellent options.

The first thing that you need to do is to warm up for 15 minutes and during the last 5 minutes perform 30 second sprints to increase your heart rate. When the 30 minutes time period starts, maintain an intensive pace to keep your heart rate at the maximum.

After 10 minutes, if your heart monitor has a lap function activate that to measure average heart rate. If you don't have that function in your monitor, you will have to record the heart beat every minute and take the average yourself at the end. This is your lactate threshold.

These two variables can help you in the determination of the intensity training zones suitable for your fitness objective.

Intensity Zones

As a fitness trainer, I know the importance of intensity zones and training with different levels of intensity to accomplish different objectives. The best way that you can determine your optimum intensity zone is from own experience and training feedback. This is known as the Perceived Level of Exertion. This can help you determine your heart rate training without a monitor.

Sometimes, during HRT, you can opt for a more rigorous pace in order to build up your aerobic capacity. The rate at which your heart pumps blood can help you to identify which energy system is dominant at specific periods of time. This is when the maximum heart rate and target heart rate become an advantage. Following are the intensity training zones which are compiled based on the percentage of the target heart rate.

1) 50% - 60% = Low Intensity

It is ideal for burning calories without stressing your body and causing injury. If you are on a low calorie diet and looking to gain muscles with maximum calorie loss this is a great zone to train in.

2) 60% - 70% = Fat-Burning Zone

This is one of the most misunderstood training zones. People think that when you are at 60 or 70 percent of your target heart rate, all the calories that you burn come from the fat. That is partly correct as only 65% of the calories come from fat and the others from the muscle mass.

3) 70% - 80% = Aerobic Zone

In this zone, the intensity of the workout increases and you burn more calories per minute. According to an estimate 45% of the calories burned during this zone come from fat. But due to more calorie loss, the overall impact on the fat loss is tremendous and if you add resistance training to it, you will not lose the muscles.

4) 80% - 90% = Anaerobic Zone

Once you reach 80% you will venture into the glycolytic and ATP-CP zones, so your relative heart rate will reach maximum or close to it and you will lose more calories per minute. The most interesting thing about this zone is that the longer you sustain a higher heart rate the longer it will take your body to recover by slowing down. This means that your body will continue to burn energy and calories to recover and the metabolism will remain high even after the training.

5) 90% - 100% = Maximal Zone

This is the training zone that experienced athletes choose. This equivalent to running all out and is used mostly in the interval training or HIIT training. In this zone, you have to apply excessive exertion over your body for intermediate lengths of times. It's not a training zone that most people will choose because it causes extreme exertion and even injury.

High Intensity Cardio

After several years of training athletes and fitness enthusiasts, I can confirm a general fact. Everyone wants to lose body fat. In most cases any effective cardiovascular exercise can help you burn excessive body fat if you perform it with consistent moderate to high intensity for more than 20 minutes. However, this is a fat loss method usually prevalent among the beginner fitness enthusiasts.

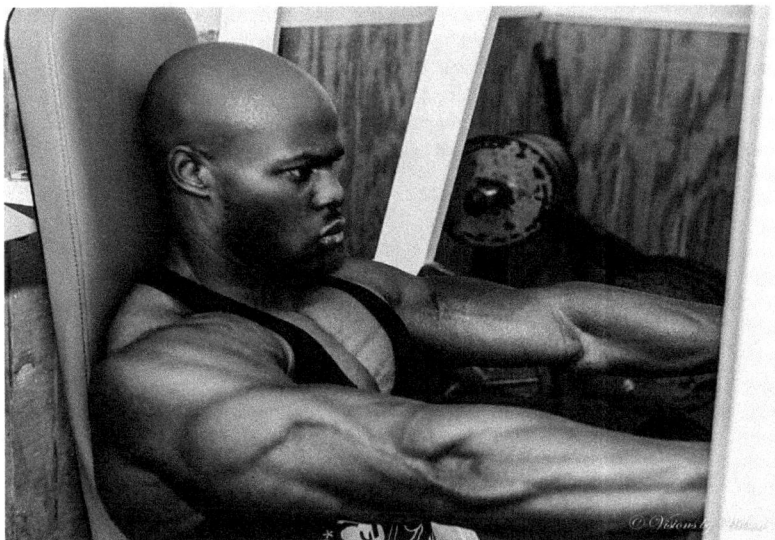

More advanced cardio practitioners prefer the strength training more commonly referred to as High Intensity Training (HIT) or conditioning. It is basically an off-shoot of the cardio strength training philosophy. The basic goal in HIT is to reach a point where you experience maximum muscular fatigue. This is the point where you cannot continue with the exercise or training. During HIT, the trainee should maintain perfect form and technique in each set, which means that the primary muscles involved in the exercise should be pushed to the limit of failure or at least close to that. This approach holds true for the cardiovascular training or conditioning as well.

The goal of HIT is to perform at such a high intensity level that your body starts burning calories in low amount of time. In order for HIT to be effective, you will need to maintain a progressive approach. This means that you will need to start on a specific level and build your stamina from that. Once a baseline has been identified and established, the next step would be to gradually increase your incline, resistance, speed and time.

The main objective of the HIT is to maintain a heart rate at a high percentage of your maximum predicted heart rate. In order to achieve that, you will need to provide maximum recovery time to your body.

Interval Training

Interval training is extremely effective for fat loss and for enhancing your cardio conditioning. With interval training, you lose more calories while stimulating your metabolism to a greater degree. You must have heard that low intensity training is effective for weight loss but it may not be the best option when it comes to fat burning. Interval training might be more challenging than low intensity workouts but it offers far greater advantages, which are explained below.

1) Interval training burns more calories than low intensity training and burns more fat in a shorter period of time.
2) It stimulates your metabolism even after the training has finished and your body continues to burn calories and fat for a long period of time post-workout.
3) In interval training, you work out at a high speed which can aid you if you are training for a sport or if you are an athlete.
4) Interval training should be done at least twice a week but no more than three times a week as it is an advance and challenging form of cardio which requires a longer recovery period. Interval training sessions can last from 5 to 30 minutes depending upon your fitness level and style of training.

How to Do Interval Training?

Interval training is based on one simple concept: go fast and then go slow. Then repeat. It is as simple as that. But this simple formula can be customized with different variations and strategies that will enable you to take full advantage of the workout. Interval training can be performed almost on every cardiovascular machine such as the treadmill, elliptical trainer, stationary bike and the Stairmaster.

Types of Interval Training

The variations of interval training that you can employ to achieve your fitness objective are truly endless. Here, I have listed different types of interval training that you can use to power your fitness routine.

1) Aerobic Training

It is a convenient and beneficial way to improve your aerobic conditioning while burning fat. It can also help you build up your endurance and can act as an introductory phase before starting hard-core interval training. This type of training involves working out for long periods with shorter work periods. Workout periods are generally 2-4 minutes long, in which you have to continue at a challenging pace, followed by a rest period of 30 seconds. The basic concept is that the shorter the rest periods, the tougher the workout will be.

2) Maximum High-Intensity Intervals

This type of interval training is very high intensity and is extremely effective for weight and fat loss. In this type of workout, you push your body to the maximum limit, which allows your body to perform faster and recover in a short amount of time. This type of maximum-effect training sends powerful signals to the metabolism increasing the growth hormones that are released in the blood stream. This process directly leads to the process initiation of fat burning. Maximum intervals are shorter than aerobic intervals, with a performance period of 30 seconds of maximal effort and then a subsequent recovery period of 30 seconds.

3) Sub-Maximal High Intensity Intervals

These types of workout sessions are expedient for fat loss and increasing your cardio conditioning. They are somewhat similar to the maximal interval style of training. The only difference is that instead of pushing yourself to the absolute limits, you workout at a pace that is a little lower than your maximum energy threshold. This allows you to work out for longer periods of time while still keeping your intensity levels high.

4) Near-Maximal Interval Training

This is a unique form of interval training that combines the aerobic interval training with the maximal interval training. This allows you to work at near peak levels for longer periods of time. In this type of training, you work at a pace that is a little short of your complete potential. It still maintains the intensity levels and allows you to challenge yourself for longer periods which lead to more fat loss and muscle gains.

High Intensity Interval Training (HIIT)

High Intensity Interval Training (HIIT) has become a popular way to burn more fat effectively. It is basically a training idea in which a trainee starts from a low intensity and gradually increases the moderate intensity level to high intensity levels. HIIT can be applied in various exercises like running or squatting. It depends on which part of the body you need to sculpt. You can target a particular body part by increasing your aerobic and anaerobic endurance capabilities while burning more fat.

If you compare the bodies of a world class runner and a world class sprinter, you will be amazed at the sprinter's body, which resembles the chiseled body of the Greek Adonis with powerful arms and chiseled quads and legs. These different body types point to the same fact that not all types of cardio are similar, which is why it is inherent that you make a correct choice based on your objective.

Recent researches state that people who participate in a steady state cardio for a period of 30 minutes showed a consistent weight loss and a loss of 0.3% of body fat. In contrast to that, people who did High-Intensity Interval Training for 20 minutes lost the same amount of weight but a whopping 2 percent loss in body fat.

It is no hidden fact that excessive aerobic activity without giving your body reasonable time to recover can lead to decreased levels of testosterones, increased cortisol production, weakened immune system and difficulty to gain muscles and any hope of hypertrophy. It doesn't mean that you cannot enhance your muscle mass development with cardio conditioning. You just have to be smart about it. You must have heard a thousand times that the conventional way to lose fat and gain muscle is to do cardio. Science tells us that this is in fact, not the case. Steady-rate cardio reduces your body's ability to absorb glucose after training. This happens because cardio can immobilize the GLUT4 transport system, which allows the translocation of insulin regulated glucose into the cells. It further causes the mTOR pathway to shut down which limits the hypertrophy to regulate muscle growth. When this happens, your body starts burning the same amount of muscles as fats, which is the last thing that a bodybuilder wants.

HIIT can help you achieve maximum muscle gains and fat loss by practicing a burst of massive cardio outputs followed by accurately timed recovery periods. Research has shown that HIIT can enhance the 24-hour Mitochondrial Biogenesis which is basically the formation of the new energy producing cells. It also helps to increase the concentration of Miliofiber nuclei which boosts the content of muscle fibers. Recent studies have shown that people, who performed at least 12 weeks of HIIT, reported a substantial decrease in body fat in the abdominal trunk and visceral area without changing their diet and nutrient intake.

The Universality of Tabata

Tabata was first introduced by the Japanese HIIT researcher Izumi Tabata. It generally consists of performing an all-out activity for 20 seconds and then resting for 10 seconds and then repeating the sequence for a total of 4 minutes. One of the most famous Tabata workouts consists of 20 seconds of all out cycling flowed by 10 seconds of low intensity cycling. This sequence is repeated for a total of four minutes for maximum VO2 capacity. Since VO2 max is considered to be the best indicator of an athlete's cardiovascular endurance and their aerobic fitness, Tabata was a game changer in the fitness industry.

Employing HIIT for Muscle Gains

When it comes to the process of gaining muscles, timing is everything. The best thing about HIIT is that it can be tweaked depending upon your preference and fitness objective. The first thing that you need to consider is how to space your workouts. The most important thing to consider is that you must time your HIIT at least 1 hour before your weight training to amplify the mitochondrial biogenesis, the benefits of which, I explained earlier.

The next thing that will affect your HIIT is volume. According to research, higher-rep, strength–endurance training best complements your HIIT sessions when they are performed on the same day. However, you must be careful not to incorporate HIIT into your daily fitness routine. It directly affects your central nervous system which takes approximately 48 hours to recover. This will result in training overflow (overtraining) which will subsequently lead to metabolic stress and mechanical tension.

HIIT can be performed in a number of ways, but to reach the maximum anaerobic levels, reach as close as you can to the maximum power output for 30 seconds, followed by a rest period of four minutes. This cycle should be repeated for at least 4-6 times thrice a week. Keep in mind that during your HIIT sessions, don't focus your mind on speed. Instead, enhance your rate of force production and resistance. The lower cadence will provide you increased level of testosterones which will aid in the muscle development.

CrossFit

The growing popularity of CrossFit has convinced a lot of people to try it. There's however, a lot to CrossFit than just wearing long socks and doing pull-ups. CrossFit was created by Coach Greg Classman to help people develop increased work capacity across board time and modal domains. It was engineered to target multiple fitness attributes at the same time. CrossFit helps you develop strength at varying levels of intensity.

In a beginner CrossFit class, you will experience what is known as Workout of the Day (WOD), which will incorporate a met-con or metabolic conditioning session. In a met-con, the goal is to include as many rounds/reps as you can in a specific period of time. The movements, rounds and reps always vary with the workout so you never know what to expect. One day, you will be doing burpees, kettle bell swings and box jumps and the next day, you could be doing pull-ups. But the concept of CrossFit goes beyond that. One of the best things about it; is that it doesn't always require a coach or even a special gym.

Difference between a Commercial Gym and CrossFit

Instead of a maze of exercise machines and rows upon rows of weights and fitness equipments, you will find that you need a smaller array of barbells, lifting platforms, rings, climbing ropes and bumper plated to complete your CrossFit session. It provides you with the ability to customize your workout based on your objective and even your mood. During CrossFit sessions, you can lift as much as you want as it allows complete freedom in personal fitness training. It will make you fitter, stronger and more athletic and mobile.

What Should You Expect From CrossFit?

Expect yourself to be challenged by CrossFit. Many people start the CrossFit regime thinking that it will be easier than intense training, but they end up performing movements and variations of exercises they have never even heard of. CrossFit expends more energy during the session which can be challenging at the start. It can sometimes depend on your coach. Good fitness facilities will employ coaches that have proper certifications. However, if you are unsure about putting your trust in certifications, feel free to ask about their background and specializations.

Core Training

The best way to gain serious mass is to develop a strong core. Core strength is the secret to building muscle mass and to grow massive proportions. It is essential if you want to experience stability and independence while moving muscles. Bones in a human body provides structure and the muscles pull on the bones at several angles, generating the force which enables us to move. It is one of the most important muscle groups in our body. If you don't have a strong core, you are at a constant threat of injuries.

The core is basically the constituent of five body parts namely, rectus abdominis (six packs), the oblique, the back extensors, the lower head of the latisimusdorsi (wings of the back), small spinal muscles (multifids muscles), transverse abdominis, glutes etc. All of these muscles work in accord to stabilize the body in movement as well as stability.

A strong core means that your body will be able to handle any shock and injury during joint movement in a better way. During every twist and turn, the muscles are at constant work to make microscopic adjustments to your body. Even in the simple movement of raising your hand, you will experience a fraction of a movement in the trunk of your body. All movements originate from your core. So if you want to lift in the gym, the initial step is to strengthen your core.

Core Training

Most of the standing exercises demand the most movement from your core muscle structure. If you are partial to exercising while being seated or lying down, you are making your core lazy. If you are lifting heavy with substantial weights and a good form, then you are on the right path, because this is best way to make your core strong. However, not every fitness program incorporates ancillary core training. Therefore, in order to include effective core workouts in your fitness program, you can consider other exercises such as anti-flexion, anti-extension and anti-rotation.

Anti-flexion exercises require you to resist the weights that attempt to pull your spine into flexion, which means that when your body extends itself to lift the weight, the excess weight causes your spine to bend in a round shape. Your job is to not let it bend and keep it in straight and perfect form. Dead lift is a great example of an anti-flexion exercise.

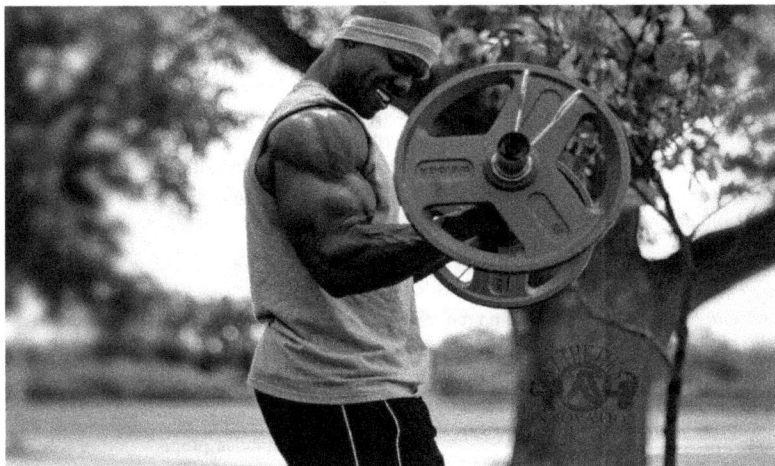

Anti-extension exercises are those that prevent in the extension or stretching of the spine while lifting a heavy load. The main goal of this exercise is the complete opposite of anti-flexion.

During an anti-rotation exercise your main job is to resist a force that will otherwise attempt to rotate your body. It can happen during an exercise which is done with a weight held on only one side of the body.

Better Form

Core training can have numerous benefits if you are an athlete, as it provides stability and an enhanced range of motions that allow you to properly perform movement patterns which would otherwise be difficult or impossible for you to perform. With a strong core, you will realize that you can lift a weight that was once quite challenging for you. It can subsequently decrease your chances of getting hurt.

If you are suffering from bad form during body building, the training processes can become excruciatingly difficult. With a strong core, you can defy the weakness and tightness of muscles by changing directions and accelerating your motions. A strong core means strong muscle groups, which prevent sprains, strains and tears. Remember that a human body is a system of intricate processes and the core is at the epicenter of it. In body building, a strong core will enable you to lift heavy loads with less stiffness and the immunity against muscle and joint injuries.

5×5 Training

The 5×5 training was specifically designed to deal with the common problems of mass development and weight plateaus and periodization while increasing strength. The 5×5 training was tailor-made to hit the muscles hard at least three times a week and then allow the body to heal and recover itself for the remaining period of time. It was initially designed for athletes as a strength training program but later, people observed that if you continue a sufficient caloric intake with the 5×5 training, you can see an increase in muscle mass.

However, if your body is not used to dealing with maximum loads and weights, then it might have a hard time coping up with the high volume and high intensity workout routine and your body will have a hard time recovering from the training.

The specialty of the 5×5 training is periodization, which means that you have to constantly change the program as you progress through it to promote the increase in muscle mass by changing the stimuli. It is quite easy to over-train during a 5×5 training due to the high intensity of the program. Therefore, you will need to prep yourself properly before starting the 5×5 training program.

Prep Yourself

The preparation time usually lasts from 4-6 weeks. During the first week, listen to the warning signs from your body and keep the training on the easier side so that you can get accustomed to the fast and hard pace that this training program requires. The most important thing that you need to ascertain is which weights to choose.

During the first week, you can perform a total of 5sets with 5 repetitions. After the first week, if you have successfully completed all your sets and reps, you will need to bump the weight from 5 to 10 pounds. But if you consider it to be too high, gradually increase the weights with moderation.

After the prep and stabilizing week, you will enter the third phase that is most commonly known as the peak phase. For the first two weeks into the peak phase, you will drop your sets and the rep combination to a 3×3 set-up. This will allow your body to push the set harder than before. Also, I suggest that you perform the squats for not more than two times a week, as the legs take more time to recover after such intensive lifting.

During these last few weeks, you will mostly concentrate on gradually increasing the weights and pushing yourself to the next level. Ideally, you should be able to break all previous weight records by the end of the peak phase. In the final weeks of the 5×5 training, you can take down the sets to one or two workouts.

German Volume Training

German Volume Training in most fitness circles is known as GVT. It is a training system that has been used by weightlifters, athletes and powerlifters to reach new fitness levels, build muscle mass, and break mass and weight plateaus. It first became popular in 1996. If you have been in the muscle building game for a while, then you might have come across several muscle building techniques such as pyramid training, reverse pyramid training, partial drop sets and many more. But GVT is one of the simplest training programs to follow. It simply consists of 10 sets of 10 reps in total. This super-easy training program is also quite effective to boost muscle and mass build-up.

Most of the body builders over-complicate things where training exercises are concerned, but GVT is effective because of the volume of work that you do in a single rep. Your only objective during a GVT is to complete 10 sets of 20 reps (100 reps in total) while using the same weights. See the chart below to help you understand the German volume Training Program.

Selecting Your Split

If you are a beginner, then a three day split will work well for you. It is an intense training program due to the high volume. However, you will be allowed rest days between the training days. The following training schedule will ensure maximum muscle boost as you will concentrate on a single muscle group in a single day.

- Day 1. Bench-press day
- Day 2. Rest
- Day 3. Squat day
- Day 4. Rest
- Day 5. Deadlift day
- Day 6. Rest
- Day 7. Rest or restart cycle

More experienced muscle builders can also focus on more than one muscle group per day, followed by mass building splits, but the high stress schedule is often too tough for beginners.

Selecting Your Exercise

In a single day, you will be concentrating on just one exercise which you have to complete in a 10×10 format per body part. Choosing an exercise is a very crucial part of this training program because you have to make sure that you select one that will boost maximum muscle building. The main objective of the German training program is to cause stimulation of the cells and causing them to swell. Therefore, combine the best types of exercises and then implement on them. For example, squats and bench-press allow the best multi-joint movement which results in enhanced metabolic stress and anabolic responses.

Choosing the Weight

This is also an important variable because if you choose an extremely high or low weight, the whole training session will be ineffective. Thus, you have to choose a weight that is at least 60% of your one-rep max also known as 1RM, which is basically the weight that you will be able to sustain for 20 reps without failure. This weight might feel a bit light for the first couple of sets, but as the collective fatigue sets in, you will find it difficult to reach the end of the workout. The most important thing to remember is not to use set-extending techniques. When you find that you can't complete the set, rest.

Rest Intervals

You should pre-determine your rest periods before starting the GVT session. The most common rest period is 90 seconds which can be maintained using a stopwatch. If you don't strictly keep to the rest schedules, the effectiveness of the overall GVT session will decrease. By limiting yourself to a rest period of 90 seconds, you will allow your muscle to rebound after the fatigue accumulates and sets in.

- **Set 1:** 185 pounds for 10 reps, rest 90 sec.
- **Set 2:** 185 pounds for 10 reps, rest 90 sec.
- **Set 3:** 185 pounds for 10 reps, rest 90 sec.
- **Set 4:** 185 pounds for 10 reps, rest 90 sec.
- **Set 5:** 185 pounds for 9 reps, rest 90 sec.
- **Set 6:** 185 pounds for 8 reps, rest 90 sec.
- **Set 7:** 185 pounds for 7 reps, rest 90 sec.
- **Set 8:** 185 pounds for 7 reps, rest 90 sec.
- **Set 9:** 185 pounds for 6 reps, rest 90 sec.
- **Set 10:** 185 pounds for 6 reps, rest 90 sec.

Supplementary Exercises

German Volume Training starts with the primary exercises done for 10 sets which are subsequently followed by complimentary exercises done from different angles with an addition of 3-8 reps. You can include two to more secondary exercises based on your experience and fitness level.

HST Program

Hypertrophy-specific training (HST) was designed by using the physiological principles of hypertrophy that were systematically organized into a mechanical method of inducing hypertrophy. The research behind hypertrophy training is rooted in the mechanisms and stimuli for muscle cell hypertrophy. However, applying these principles into developing and boosting muscles can be complicated and traditional training techniques cannot be applied to induce muscle hypertrophy. Here are some basic hypertrophy principles which allowed Bryan Haycock to develop the HST workout techniques practiced by a variety of lifters worldwide.

Mechanical Load

It is the most important variable to induce muscle hypertrophy. This mechanism includes the MAPk/ERK, satellite cells, growth mechanism and calcium levels. However, HST is not limited to these variables. It depends equally on the muscle fiber types that participate in muscle growth when they are exposed to excess weight loads. This is in direct contrast to the notion that you have to work your muscles to failure before the muscle fibers have any chance of growth.

By an extension of this variable, the effectiveness of an HST workout cannot be calculated based on the amount of fatigue. Rather, the HST workout directs the bodybuilder to focus on enhancing the mechanical stress brought upon by heavy loads which causes micro trauma and muscle mass development.

Acute Vs. Chronic Frequency

For an HST program to be effective, stimulus must be applied with consistent frequency to ensure increased hypertrophy. It is in direct contrast to the principle of applying random and acute assaults on your muscle cells and tissues to boost muscular integrity. The major drawback of taking a week to rest is that the acute responses of the loaded muscle will increase the protein synthesis, prostaglandins, IGF-1 levels, and mRNA levels, which return back to normal after 36 hours.

Therefore, if you spend two days for mass development and half a week to recover in an anti-symbiotic state, the recovery will take place even if you re-load your muscles within 48 hours. The remaining time will allow your body to replace and balance nitrogen retention without any more additions.

Progression

This principle of the HST training states, that the mechanical loading of the muscles must progress gradually. Normally, a human body prefers homeostasis, which means the loading of the muscles in a particular manner which becomes ineffective when stimulated as an adaptive response. In order to keep this adaptive response working, you must increase the weights throughout the weight cycle. This allows the tissues to become resistant and adaptive. This adaptation can occur during a Repeated Bout Effect or a Rapid Training Effect in as little as 48 hours.

Strategic Conditioning

This principle states that we must practice predetermined periods to rest and recover our muscles and to become de-conditioned to the loads used during the HST training. Strategic conditioning is the most probable consequence of the principle of progression. After progression, you can either increase the load or decrease the conditioning. As the muscle becomes sensitive to the change in load; therefore, it generates a hypertrophic effect when you increase the load from the previous session. This can also allow you to reach your maximum voluntary strength and can prove to be favorable for builders who experience sudden growth stagnation.

Part 2: Muscle Building Routines

When it comes to muscle building, there are several methods, techniques and preferences which depend on the builder's goals. It doesn't matter if your overall goal is to improve your health, fitness level, appearance or a combination of these. There is no shortage of muscle building techniques to help you achieve these objectives. However, finding the best one can be difficult as you might not know which one will work best for you unless you try it out. However, the following routines can help you figure out your category requirement.

3 Day Full Body Routine

This workout routine has to be practiced for just three days a week. Each training day is followed by a rest day and the third workout is followed by at least 1 to 2 days of rest. This routine is usually followed by beginners who start by full body workouts. It is ideal for beginners because it allows you to become familiar with the exercises by repetitions throughout the week. It also aids you to gradually develop muscle strength by lifting light loads first, allowing the muscles to quickly repair themselves before the next workout.

During the first few weeks of this routine; beginners will experience greater gains if they train less. This is also known as the beginner's gain period which is your body's natural response when it adapts to exercises. This will allow you to gradually increase the volume and frequency of the weights and reps in the coming weeks.

4-Day Split

The next possible step up, from the 3-day split is the 4-day split which is performed by intermediate lifters. There are several variations of this training program focusing on upper body workouts first, followed by the lower body workouts on the following day. After that, you take a rest day to give your body the time to recover. Then the whole process is repeated all over. However, you will have the choice to take a day or two off to recover.

5-Day Split Routine

The 5-day split is a workout routine that can be practiced by experienced to intermediate bodybuilders. There are several routines that make you train 7 days a week or even twice per day which amounts to a total of 14 workouts per week. However, after training for a number of years, you reach your maximum muscle level and strength and this routine can help you maintain your muscle mass. This can also help you, if it has become a lot harder for you to add gains or grow additional muscle. This workout can be followed by increasing the volume and allowing your body time to recover for a day or two to stimulate muscle growth.

Part 3: Strength Training

As a bodybuilder, when you lift, repetitions matters a lot. But one other thing that can help you reach maximum strength and muscle gain is the negative portion of the lifts, also known as the eccentric half of the lift.

On the whole, the major focus of your workout is to lift the weights, which allows your muscles to shorten. Whichever body part you are targeting during an exercise, will shorten concentrically. Thus, lifting a weight is also known as positive rep training.

In contrast to this, when you lower the weights, your muscles experience something called negative training as it causes your muscle to lengthen or extend, because the external resistance is greater than the applied force. Numerous studies have shown that if you want to develop greater volume of muscle mass, you should focus more on eccentric training rather than just concentric training. The most important reason for that is that the longer your muscles are under tension and stress, the more protein will be synthesized, which will increase the insulin levels.

Eccentric strength training can also help you increase type II muscle fibers which have the greatest potential for muscle hypertrophy. This allows your muscles to feel less fatigued, thus requiring less energy to lift greater volume of weights. All of these variables add up to one single fact, a direct increase in size as well as strength. Most of the body builders want to get big as well as strong and while the initial increase in heavy stimulus may work on the surface, you will soon face the quandary of block training or linear periodization. For consistent gains, it is important to understand the science behind strength training and how you can use it to develop muscle mass.

A Beginner's Guide to Strength Training

Every time you lift a weight, your strength and hypertrophy will be challenged. But the degree to which that is possible depends upon how each adaptation is stimulated by systematically arranging the training variables. These variables can include volume, intensity, and type of workout or training phase. In short, becoming stronger requires that your muscles increase in size by experiencing load intensity. In truth, a human body will adapt more successfully to overcome a single demand rather than working on multiple demands at the same time. This is because when you lift to gain size, it is quite different as compared to when you are lifting to gain strength.

Nevertheless, we cannot ignore the fact that the stronger we are, the more we will be able to lift. This can give you a long-term body building advantage.

Is Size And Strength Correlated Or Codependent?

After spending a few weeks focusing on your strength training, you will feel stronger in the muscle building portion of your fitness routine. This increased strength will allow you to lift heavier weights, thus increasing the overall volume of your training. Your body will be able to handle more weight in any multi-joint exercises.

As a beginner, you may experience fast gains in the initial few months of body building. However, these gains will slow down or come to a complete halt after some time. A short term solution would be to add more volume, exercises, forced reps and other advance training techniques like negative training. But you will notice that soon these techniques will stop yielding results and your mass development will plateau again. This is where strength training comes in.

Training specifically for strength will lead you to perform exercise combinations and variables which you can alter based on your level of training. These variables are the choice of exercises, order of exercises, number of sets, recovery time between sets and the resistance level. Your body's reaction to resistance training will be different, depending upon your approach. After the initial break-in period of 4-6 weeks, your muscle fibers will go through the process of adaptation and subsequently grow larger at both intracellular and neurological levels.

More Weight, Less Reps

When you are training to gain mass, the most important thing is to follow moderate rep sets which have a direct effect on training volume. In order to build strength, you will have to train with heavier weights, which will necessitate low reps. The first exercise of the day after warm up should be a pyramid of increasing weights. The secret to success is to stop the training before muscle failure. It is quite easy to determine your working weights from strength training. Choose a weight that falls within 80-90% of your 1RM which might seem heavier than usual, but trust me, it is perfect for 4-8 reps that fall between the 10-20 range.

The Importance of Assistance Exercises

The biggest mistake you can make while choosing assistance exercises for your strength training program is to follow the conventional process by which you choose complimentary exercises for your bodybuilding routine. If you do that, you can overwhelm and stress your nervous system by employing a high intensity rather than the high volume approach that is consistent in strength training. Ideally, assistance exercises are chosen for their ability to target our weak points and improve our main lifts. For some lifters, it can be the bottom of the lift while for others it could be the locking-out point.

Extend Your Rest Periods

You may have wondered sometimes about why experienced bodybuilders take extended rest periods. The primary reason for that is that the heavier the weights are; the more stress you are exerting on your muscles and the more time it will take for them to recover. When you are lifting heavy weights, the body directly derives the energy from the anaerobic metabolism, which is also known as the ATP-PC (Adenosine triphosphate-phosphocreatine) system. This metabolism provides the energy surge which is required to lift heavy weights or perform any explosive movements but only for short periods of time. This pathway system can require at least a 3-minute recovery period.

Now that you know the basics of building strength, you can apply this knowledge during your next training session. Remember to build your strength by concentrating on a main lift per training day. Keep the volume low to counter intensive training, after which your body will become primed to build more muscle mass.

Chapter#3: Muscle Building Variables

Is Cluster Training Important To Increase Mass Volume?

Cluster training can increase the force production and can be a great help in developing mass consistently. Cluster sets are intra-set with rest periods to allow the body to sustain more weights, reps and tonnage during the workouts. The built-in sets can be manipulated and depend on your desired outcome.

You may think that it sounds a lot like rest and pause training. It is somewhat similar to it but the main difference is that it doesn't have a set load and a pre-dictated volume. On the other hand, in cluster training, you have a set volume and the load and its main focus is not acquiring training fatigue but rather to decrease the overall metabolic fatigue formed by the "no rest" sets. Cluster training should be performed during your main lifts of the day, for example bench press, incline press and military press. After those, you can continue with your secondary workouts, like triceps extensions and side raises.

Outdoor Activities for Muscle Building

If you are thinking about taking advantage of the weather and training outside, it can help you to supplement your strength and muscle building program with a couple of outdoor activities that can be customized based on your fitness pace and needs. If you want to see fast results, you must remember that these activities are just complimentary to the muscle building exercises and they can never replace them where muscle building is concerned. However, these athletic activities will improve your gains; enhance your conditioning and shed a small percentage of the body fat in the whole process. Some of the most common outdoor activities for mass development are given below.

Sprinting

It is an explosive science that stresses your anaerobic levels and trains the muscles to respond to the fast twitch muscle fibers that are controlled by the high threshold motor units. These motor units are the primary variable in the heavy lifting and low rep during short duration workouts. Sprinting is also useful for increasing the metabolic rate by excessive post-exercise oxygen consumption, that burns fat even after the workout is done.

Loaded Carriers

Fireman's carriers, atlas carriers, overhead carriers and farmer's carriers only require a couple of dumb bells or plates and can easily be done outside. They are very helpful in developing mass volume in the shoulder, triceps, and forearm area. The main difference between sprinting and loaded carriers is that you are covering the same amount of distance but with added weight that subsequently increases your grip strength causing your body to work overtime. From a hypertrophy standpoint, these types of exercises allow the bodybuilder to respond well to the endurance training.

Prowler Pushing

Prowler pushing combines the attributes of weighted sprinting and lower body stress workouts. It helps increase and improves the lower body's form and technique. This form of exercise uses the physical variables to create the highest force output and velocity, which enables proper joint alignment for mechanical efficiency.

Lunges

Dumbbell or barbell-loaded walking lunges are often overlooked by bodybuilders who are looking to increase mass. However, you shouldn't ignore the advantages of loaded lunges on the hypertrophic response of the body when you train your body under stress for extended time periods. This high endurance workout can kill your cardio endurance but don't let it stop you from finishing your workout as the quad muscles will be burning by the end of it if you maintain good form throughout your workout.

Developing Mass Muscles Naturally

Gaining muscles without harmful chemicals and steroids is possible. The following muscle and mass development tips can help you combat fast metabolism and achieve the gains that you are looking for.

1) It doesn't matter which training or workout program you are following. Keep the duration of your training session under an hour. Concentrate in keeping your intensity and stress levels high rather than extending your workout.
2) Focus on eating consistently. Don't miss out on meals. If you are unfortunate to have a fast metabolism, it can hinder the process of mass development by digesting the food quickly and burning the calories before your body can metabolize the nutrients into muscle fibers. Therefore, break down your eating schedule into eating 3-4 high caloric meals throughout the day.
3) Supplements can be quite beneficial where mass development is concerned, but don't rely on them completely. Be very careful when you are selecting supplements. Make sure that they don't have any harmful chemicals and synthetic ingredients.
4) Don't over-exert your body or over train.
5) Understand the basic concept of caloric surplus. It's not just about increasing the amount of food that you eat. Re-evaluate your diet and consume food that is rich in protein to help the process of muscle building. If you are not used to eating large

quantities of food, you will feel a little uncomfortable with the high food intake at first, but your body will soon adjust, due to the high energy consumption during your training sessions.

6) Keep your eye on the prize and focus your mind on progress. The more volume you put in your training sessions, the more results you will see. Focus on increasing the weights and reps. Break your stress threshold and push yourself to the limit.

7) Change your rep combination every other week. This periodic change will help you to avoid plateaus. If your body becomes accustomed to a weight and rep combination, mass development will stop, as your body will become adapted to the routine.

Efficient Warm-Ups Can Maximize Your Workouts

As a hard gainer, it is my firm belief that the warm process can make or break your whole workout routine. Some bodybuilders have a misconception that warm-ups actually mean getting "warm". In actuality, warm-up is the time that you should use to get ready, in order to perform to your maximum capacity. The warm up session usually consists of a 10 minute stretching session or a mild run on the treadmill.

The main objective of the warm-up session is to lengthen your muscles and enhance the force-couple relationship. This will ensure a high performance and injury-free workout. Here are some of the approaches that I prefer in a warm-up session to get the blood going.

1) Use a foam roller to actively target your trigger points. Your body will be able to move easily. Foam rolling does hurt but not more than rehab or surgery.

2) Increasing the length of your muscles by static stretching can increase your risk of injury by 30%. Therefore, I normally discourage this method. I propose that you focus more on dynamic stretching which allows the muscles to lengthen naturally. You can do that by performing a couple of sets of chest and hamstring curls for quads.

3) Perform a single exercise that energizes your central nervous system and creates an optimal connection between the mind and the muscle. Slow underhanded pull-ups and sissy squats are some of the examples to target your muscles for better performance.

Is Resistance Training Helpful?

Resistance training is simply made up of exercises in which you work against the forces that hinder movement. Weightlifting is just one example of resistance training. Other exercises that fall in this category are dragging sleds, bodyweight exercises, running with parachutes and training in water or sand. It can be quite helpful in the overall mass development process. Resistance training helps you get used to the challenging weights while maintaining good form. It allows better movement patterns and breathing mechanisms.

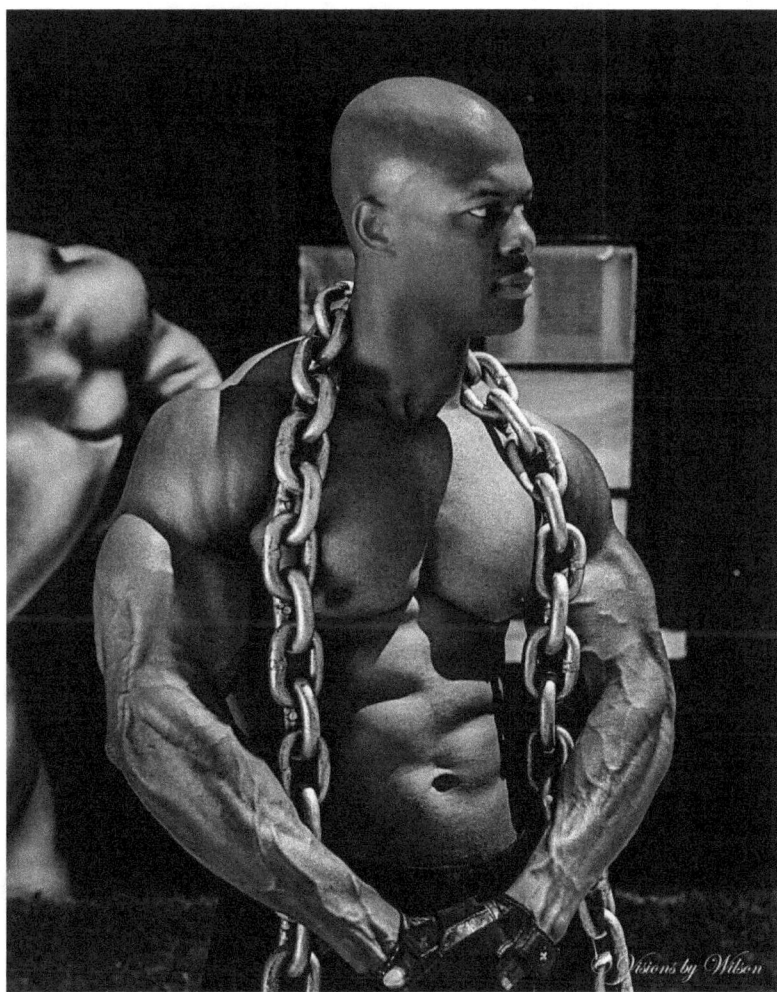

Chapter#5: Supplementation for Bodybuilders

If your goal is to increase muscle mass or strength, supplement intake is very important. It can help you get maximum impact out of your workout routines. Knowing which supplements to take, how much to take and even the correct time to take them will determine the final results of your mass development.

Types of Supplements

There are several types of muscle building supplements that can help you to enhance the lean structure of your body, increase mass volume and help the body recover after an intense workout. You must remember that each person is blessed with a different body type. Therefore, the supplements will affect each one of you in a unique way. Despite all these differences, here are some of the supplements that offer great benefits and returns in the development of muscle volume.

Creatine Monohydrate

This is a muscle building and power enhancing supplement. It has been supported by various research and studies as being a safe and effective way to increase the availability of Creatine and phosphocreatine within the muscles while maintaining sufficient amount of energy during high intensity training sessions. It can also help in recovery and in enhancing the quality of your endurance level. The recommended dose is 20 grams per day for 5-7 days, followed by a dosage of 5 grams a day.

Caffeine

Caffeine is a widely available stimulant which is used as an effective ergogenic tool to increase the endurance level during intensive workouts. However, it is better not to take a caffeine supplement before starting strength or resistance training as it has no effect on the strength variable. It can however, be of great help in reducing fatigue or in improving a lower perception of motivation and effort. The recommended dose is 150-300 milligrams which can be taken 30-60 minutes before a workout.

Branched-Chain Amino Acids (BCAAs)

If you are a body builder, you must be aware of the delicious BCAAs that help your body recover quickly after a tough workout. It also regulates protein metabolism in the body by increasing the protein synthesis levels and decreasing protein degradation. The recommended dose is 6-10 grams before or during a workout.

Citrulline Malate

It was originally introduced as an anti-fatigue supplement and is popular among heavy lifters as a performance booster. The benefits associated with CM supplements are because of the synergistic combination of L-Citrullineand Malate, which directly increases the ATP rates during the exercise and the PCr recovery rate after the workout. It has also shown increased performance during upper and lower body resistance exercises. The recommended dose is 8 grams, which can be taken approximately 60 minutes before the workout.

NO (Nitric Oxide) Boosters

Nitrate-rich foods such as beets and pomegranates are a great way to increase your nitric oxide levels. They increase the skeletal muscle blood flow which can help with post muscle soreness. They can also aid in improving hypertrophy and strength in resistance-trained bodybuilders. The recommended dose is 500 milligrams of beet juice or pomegranate juice at least an hour before your workout.

Whey Protein

Whey protein has gained popularity for being a fast digesting protein that can enhance your muscle's ability to recover and rebound after a strenuous round of exercises. It can also stimulate protein synthesis to a greater degree than other proteins such as soy, tofu and casein. A combination of fast digesting whey and slow digesting casein keeps the body in a high metabolic state for an extended period of time, all the while maintaining the protein synthesis rate, thus minimizing any muscle loss. If you are a high intensity resistance trainer, combing carbohydrates with whey protein can increase your insulin levels and the re-synthesis rate of glycogens. The recommended dose is 20-30 grams, preferably after the workout, for better mass volume.

Glutamine

This is a type of amino acid which plays an important role to recover the muscles by removing access amounts of ammonia from the body that can accumulate during an intensive training session. People who are regularly engaged in resistance training, training splits or suffer from calorie deficit in their diets can benefit from consistent intake of glutamine supplements. The recommended dose is 20-30 grams a day, 10 gram of which can be taken post-training.

Fish Oils

Fish oil supplements are an excellent source of omega-3 fatty acids, which provide a plethora of benefits to our body. In bodybuilding, fish oil supplements allow the body to go through quick stages of anti-inflammation and anti-oxidation. They also repair the microscopic tears in your muscles which are caused by the resistance training. Combining it with BCAAs and carbs will lead to greater gains in muscle mass. The recommended dose is 2 grams daily, taken during a meal.

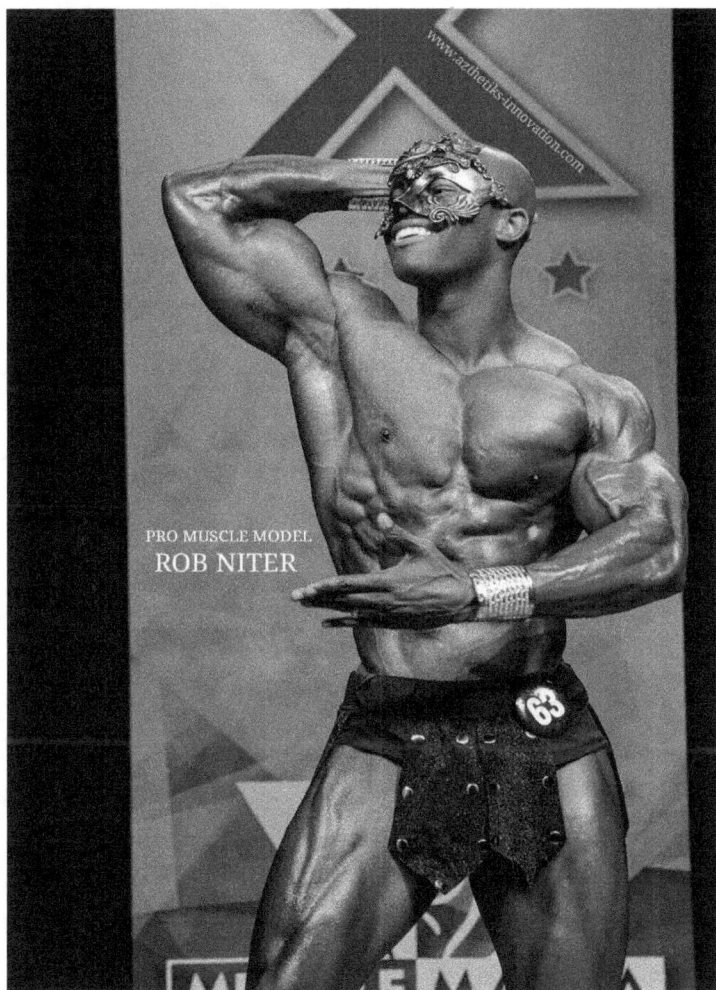

PRO MUSCLE MODEL
ROB NITER

Chapter#6: Nutrition

Nutrition is essential for growth and recovery, without which, muscle building is impossible. The most common problem that most bodybuilders face in this regard is their constantly changing bodies and their nutrient demand. A consistent increase in muscle mass means that you have to constantly tweak your diet plan. The best solution hence, is to keep track of your body's changes. Weighing yourself regularly and using body fat calipers to keep track of your muscle measurements can help you determine the overall body fat percentage. This chapter will explain every aspect of a bodybuilder's diet and how it effects the mass development.

How Can You Create a Bodybuilding Diet

Without proper nutrition, you won't be able to develop mass. It is an important part of the whole bodybuilding process. The first step in creating a perfect mass development diet is to calculate your body fat and fat free mass. You can learn how to calculate your body fat from the adjacent table.

Example of calculations of body fat, and fat free mass, using the weight as 200lb, and a body fat percentage of 21%.

Body fat Calculations:

Bodyweight:	200lbs
Body fat Percentage:	21%

The Calculations:

Step1. Bodyweight x body fat percentage = lb body fat.
(200 x 0.21 = 42 lb body fat)

Step2. Bodyweight – 42 = fat free mass (200 – 42 = 158) (This figure is the total amount of fat free mass).

Body weight:	200lbs
Body fat Percentage:	21%
Total Body fat:	42lbs
Fat Free Mass:	158lbs

After that, you will need to calculate your caloric intake that you need to consume in a day. There are several online calories calculators that you can use for this purpose. After following every instruction, if you still feel that you are not gaining weight, eat twice the amount of carbs and 1.5 times the amount of protein as you normally do, at least twice a day. If you are gaining weight but the percentages of fat and muscles are similar, try to eliminate carbs from at least the last two meals of your day. If you are losing body weight constantly, try to divide your carbohydrate intake into two for the last two meals. If the body fats drop, immediately increase your carbs intake, especially after a workout session.

Image 1

The best foods to incorporate in your diet plan are protein rich foods like meat, fish and poultry as well as legumes, nuts, seeds, dairy, eggs, grains, fruits and vegetables.

The Importance of Eating Frequently

Skipping meals can have disastrous effects on your muscle mass development. You must remember that proper and frequent nutrition is inherent to completing your daily routine tasks as well as the physical training. In order to avoid dire consequences, it is very important not to skip any meals.

It might sound appealing and convenient to you, but when you skip a meal, your body goes into a fasting mode, during which the stored body nutrients are used for energy generation. The glycogen levels in the liver and muscles become depleted and the body breaks down the protein in your muscles as an alternating source of fuel. The body starts metabolizing fat as a fighting mechanism and a massive decrease in T3 thyroid hormone occurs which can effect and lower your insulin levels. This can cause your lean muscles to shrink and become weaker.

If you don't eat frequently, your body may plunge into the starvation mode which causes muscle loss and decrease in metabolism. All of these factors lower your performance level during a workout which can have a direct effect on muscle growth.

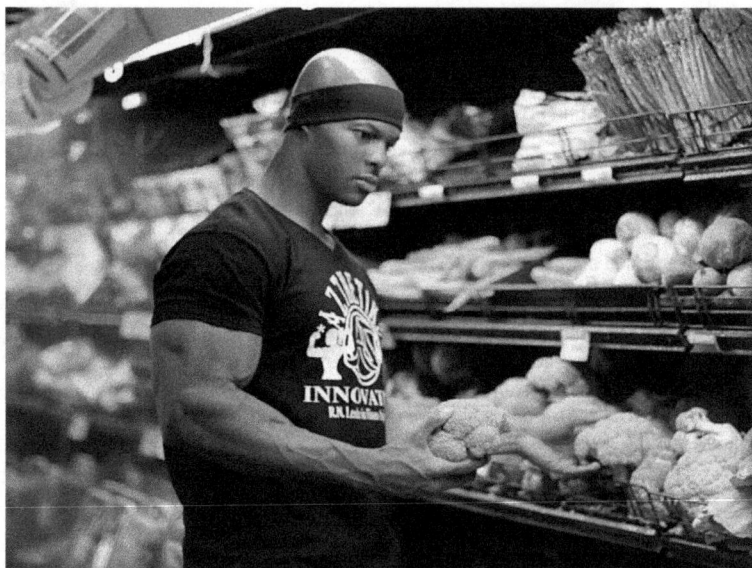

The Myth about Intermittent Fasting

Intermittent fasting has become popular enough to accumulate a cult-like following. However, there are several misconceptions about intermittent fasting that have floated around the fitness world for quite some time. Many people consider it detrimental to the growth and recovery process and associate it with an unhealthy lifestyle. But before coming to a definite conclusion, let us discuss some of the most common myths related to intermittent fasting.

Intermittent Fasting Has Limited Uses For A Limited Population

It is the complete opposite of the prevailing trend. People nowadays, find it more difficult to eat round the clock and keep track of meals all day long. Intermittent fasting is thus, easier to follow.

It Leads To Eating Disorders

Intermittent fasting doesn't lead to eating disorders like bulimia and binge eating disorder. People who practice this lifestyle simply keep track of the calorie and nutrient intake as the timing of the meal is not important. Besides this fact, eating big meals in a day means more nutrient intake per meal.

Big Evening Meals with Carbohydrates Can Result In Fat Gain

The misconception that insulin sensitivity is generally lower at night is not true. Eating carbs with evening meals will lead to carbohydrate oxidation but to think that you would gain fat in the absence of increased energy consumption is untrue.

Intermittent Fasting Leads to Muscle Loss

Just because you are not eating frequent meals doesn't mean that your body is in a catabolic mode. This eating lifestyle includes a large protein portion that can slowly digest and release amino acids. This is true that it can cause some muscle loss when de novo gluconeo-genesis activates after the liver and muscle glycogens are running low. However, if you eat large meal portions during fasting periods, this is unlikely to occur.

Are Carbohydrates Bad For You?

As a fitness trainer, people always ask me if carbs are bad for them. The answer is no, carbs are not bad for you. Carbohydrates are an energy source for the body which can be stored in the liver and muscles for energy consumption by every cell in our body. Most of the carbohydrates come from plant and animal sources. The complex carbs have a healthy amount of fiber that aids in the bowel movements and stabilize the blood sugar levels by decreasing the glycogen absorption rate in the body.

Carbohydrates also decrease cholesterol levels, thus reducing the risk for heart diseases. For those who are looking to get lean and lose fat, fibers in carbs can help you stay full much longer by curbing your appetite. However, this fact should not be ignored that high-carb intake can lead to increased glycogen levels which produce excess amounts of glucose. It is thus, inherent to eat only the fiber-rich brown variety of carbs which will decrease the risk of fat storage enzymes, and decrease the chance of gaining fat.

Final Words

This book is the amalgamation of knowledge that I have acquired during my whole life as a fitness trainer and bodybuilder. Everything mentioned in this book will help you to reach the ultimate goal of developing muscle mass and enhance your training. The workout routines and programs will have a profound effect on your body. But maintaining a proper dietary and supplementary intake is also very important.

Staying strong physically and mentally, while maintaining your motivation levels, is not an easy task. You will struggle and you will have hardships; but having the will power to not surrender, will give you strength. Continue to keep your eyes on the objective and remain focused. Remember the reasons that why you started this journey in the first place. Work for the body you want and push yourself to the absolute limits. I dedicate this book to those who want to convert to a healthier lifestyle, while in search for direction and guidance. In my years of experience, I learned that nothing is impossible and there is no challenge too great. I have seen skinny guys get ripped and gain muscle. I have watched overweight women shed excess fat when they didn't think they could. I am a living testimony to their success. I have worked tirelessly to change the lives of hundreds of people, by customizing my training programs based on their fitness level and goals. It is to my belief that I am called for the task at hand. I say to you, "NEVER give up on a dream just because of the time it will take for you to accomplish it. NEVER cower away from an obstacle just because it's easier." That's for anything in life. By following the guidelines listed in this book, you can reach your bodybuilding goals and become a sensational fitness leader for those to emulate. Thank you for inspiring me, for reading along and sharing my wisdom! Now let's go get 'em CHAMP!

FOLLOW ME:

FACEBOOK.COM/ROBNITEROFFICIAL

INSTAGRAM.COM/ROBNITER

TWITTER.COM/ROBNITER

WWW.AZTHETIKS-INNOVATION.COM

www.ingramcontent.com/pod-product-compliance
Lightning Source LLC
Chambersburg PA
CBHW060642280326
41933CB00012B/2126

* 9 7 8 1 3 7 0 8 5 0 3 3 4 *